THE CANCER FIX:
Cancer Prevention and Treatment Tips Through Lifestyle Changes

BY

DR. HENRY FOSTER

Copyright © by Henry Foster 2022. All rights reserved.

Before this document is duplicated or reproduced in any manner, the publisher's consent must be gained. Therefore, the contents within can neither be stored electronically, transferred, nor kept in a database. Neither in Part nor full can the document be copied, scanned, faxed, or retained without approval from the publisher or creator.

THE CANCER FIX: Cancer Prevention and Treatment Tips Through Lifestyle Changes 1
INTRODUCTION 4
CHAPTER ONE 8
WHAT IS CANCER? WHAT ARE ITS CAUSES? 8
  What distinguishes benign cancer from malignant cancer? 8
  What does it mean for cancer to be "locally invasive" or "metastatic"? 8
  Primary and Secondary tumors 9
  Why Does Cancer Occur? 9
  Cancer Risk Elements 10
  Cancer Genes 12
  How do genes impact cancer development? 12
  Cancer gene classifications 13
CHAPTER TWO 15
HEALTHY DIET 15
  Weight changes during cancer treatment 17
  Dietary interventions 18
  Calorie limitation 19
  Ketogenic diet/carbohydrate restriction 20
  Additional dietary strategies 21
  Which diet is best for cancer therapy? 22
CHAPTER THREE 25
FASTING 25

Increasing Sensitivity to Insulin	26
Reversing the effects of chronic diseases	26
Enhancing Autophagy	27
Improving Living Conditions While Receiving Chemotherapy	27
Increasing Immunity to Fight Cancer	28
CHAPTER FOUR	30
EXERCISE	30
What advantages does exercise provide for cancer patients?	30
Things you need to know before you exercise during cancer therapy	32
Developing your exercise regimen	32
Stretching	33
How to work out while receiving cancer therapy safely	34
How does exercise fit into a regimen for cancer rehabilitation?	36
Ask the medical staff these questions	36
CHAPTER FIVE	38
REGULAR CHECK-UPS	38
Why should you be aware of your cancer status?	39
You cannot afford to avoid cancer screening.	40
CONCLUSION	42

INTRODUCTION

Cancer is a broad collection of illnesses that can begin in practically any organ or tissue of the body. These illnesses are brought on when abnormal cells grow out of control, cross their normal boundaries to infect nearby body parts and/or spread to other organs. The latter process, known as metastasizing, is a significant contributor to cancer-related mortality. The terms "neoplasm" and "malignant tumor" are also used to describe cancer.

An estimated 9.6 million deaths, or one in every six deaths, were attributed to cancer in 2018, making it the second highest cause of death worldwide. Men are more likely to develop lung, prostate, colorectal, stomach, and liver cancer than women, who are more likely to develop breast, colorectal, lung, cervical, and thyroid cancer.

The physical, emotional, and monetary toll that cancer takes on people, families, communities, and health systems is increasing on a global scale. Large numbers of cancer patients worldwide lack access to prompt, high-quality diagnosis and treatment because many health systems in low- and middle-income nations are least equipped to handle this load. The availability of early identification, high-quality treatment, and survivorship care in nations with robust health systems has improved the survival rates of numerous cancer forms.

By altering or eliminating significant risk factors and putting into practice currently recommended evidence-based preventative methods, between 30% and 50% of cancer-related fatalities could be avoided. Through early cancer detection and patient management, the burden of cancer can also be decreased. The most economical long-term approach to the control of cancer is prevention.

The following significant risk factors can be modified or avoided to help prevent cancer:

- Do not use tobacco products, such as cigarettes or smokeless tobacco.
- keep a healthy weight.
- consume a nutritious diet rich in fruits and vegetables.
- Regular exercise
- drink in moderation
- sex should be safe.
- be immunized against the human papillomavirus and hepatitis B (HPV)
- lessen your exposure to UV rays
- limit the exposure to ionizing radiation (e.g. minimize occupational exposure, ensure safe and appropriate medical use of radiation in diagnosis and treatment)
- Avoid using solid fuels in your home to reduce indoor smoke and pollution from the city
- regular medical attention
- Some persistent infections can increase your risk of developing cancer. Chronic infections increase the risk of cancer development in people living in low- and middle-income nations.

When cancer is detected early, it is more likely to respond to appropriate treatment, increasing the likelihood of survival as well as reducing morbidity and treatment costs.

Early detection is encouraged by two different tactics:

1. Early cancer detection finds cases of the disease at the earliest possible stage.
2. The goal of screening is to locate people who have abnormalities suggestive of a particular disease or pre-cancer but who do not yet have any symptoms so that they can be quickly diagnosed and treated.

Surgery, cancer medications, and/or radiotherapy, either alone or in combination, are available as treatment options. Based on tumor kind, cancer stage, clinical, and other characteristics, a multidisciplinary team of cancer experts suggests the optimal treatment strategy. Patients' wishes should be taken into account, as well as the capabilities of the healthcare system.

A crucial part of cancer treatment is palliative care, which aims to enhance the quality of life for patients and their families. A comprehensive plan for tracking cancer recurrence and spotting new cancers, evaluating and treating the long-term side effects of cancer and/or its treatment, and services to meet the needs of cancer survivors are all included in survivorship care.

In addition to learning about some lifestyle hacks to avoid, fight, and manage cancer, this book will teach you about the various causes of cancer and how they manifest. Cancer is a fatal illness, but it doesn't have to be your demise. As we examine the illness known as cancer, take a seat back and unwind.

CHAPTER ONE
WHAT IS CANCER? WHAT ARE ITS CAUSES?

Cancer is defined as abnormal cell proliferation. Even in the face of space constraints, the availability of nutrients to other cells, or signals from the body to stop reproduction, cancer cells continue to grow quickly. In addition to not functioning properly, cancer cells frequently differ in structure from healthy cells and have the ability to spread throughout the body. Clusters of cells that are capable of uncontrollably expanding and dividing—tumors, abnormal growth of tissue—are characterized by uncontrolled cell growth.

The study of cancer and tumors is called "Oncology". When a tumor is malignant, which means it has the potential to cause harm, including death, the term "cancer" is used to describe it.

What distinguishes benign cancer from malignant cancer?
Malignant or benign tumors can both occur in the body (cancerous). It is typical for benign tumors to grow slowly and not spread. Malignant tumors have the ability to spread throughout the body, grow quickly, infiltrate neighboring normal tissues, and do great damage.

What does it mean for cancer to be "locally invasive" or "metastatic"?

Cancer is malignant because it can be "locally invasive" and "metastatic":

Locally invasive cancer: The tumor can spread "fingers" of malignant cells into the surrounding healthy tissue, invading those areas.

Metastatic cancer occurs when a tumor sends cells to tissues outside of the primary tumor.

Primary and Secondary tumors

The term "primary tumor" refers to the initial tumor, whose cells can spread throughout the body and start the development of secondary tumors in different organs. "Secondary tumors" are the name for these brand-new tumors.

Secondary tumors are created when malignant cells spread through the lymphatic or circulatory systems. A network of tiny vessels called the lymphatic system is responsible for collecting waste from cells, transporting it into larger vessels, and then directing it to lymph nodes. Eventually, lymph fluid enters the circulation.

Why Does Cancer Occur?

Cancer can have many different causes. According to scientists, the combination of numerous elements results in cancer. The contributing elements may be a person's constitutional traits, environmental influences, or genetics.

Tumors in children are treated differently than cancers in adults in terms of diagnosis, prognosis, and treatment. The likelihood of survival and the origin of the malignancy are the primary variations. While adult cancers have a survival rate of 68%, juvenile cancers have an overall five-year survival rate of roughly 80%. This difference is believed to exist because pediatric cancer responds better to treatment and children may withstand more rigorous treatment.

Stem cells, which are uncomplicated cells capable of creating different kinds of specialized cells that the body requires, frequently cause or start childhood malignancies. Typically, juvenile cancer is brought on by a random (happens by chance) cell alteration or mutation. The sort of cell that develops into cancer in adulthood is typically an epithelial cell. Body cavities and the exterior of the body are lined with epithelial cells. Environmental exposures to these cells over time can result in cancer. For this reason, adult cancers are occasionally referred to as acquired.

Cancer Risk Elements

As was previously stated, several malignancies, particularly in adults, have been linked to repeated exposures or risk factors.

Anything that could make someone more likely to contract an illness is considered a risk factor. A risk factor may weaken the body's resistance to the disease even though it may not always cause it. As potential risk factors and cancer-causing pathways, the following include:

lifestyle elements. Various lifestyle choices that may increase your risk of developing some adult malignancies include smoking, eating a lot of fat, and working with hazardous chemicals. However, most cancer patients are too young to have had any extended exposure to these lifestyle risks.

Family history, inheritance, and genetics may all play a role in some childhood malignancies. It is conceivable for a family to experience cancer in different forms more than once. In some cases, it is unclear if the illness is brought on by a genetic mutation, exposure to chemicals in the area around a family's home, a mix of these factors, or perhaps happenstance.

Certain genetic conditions. For instance, it is known that the immune system is altered by the Wiskott-Aldrich and Beckwith-Wiedemann syndromes. The immune system is a sophisticated system that guards against sickness and infection in our bodies. Cells that eventually develop and serve as an element of the immune system are created in the bone marrow. According to one idea, the stem cells in the bone marrow have flaws or defects that cause them to produce cancerous or aberrant cells when they divide to make more of them. The stem cell deficiency may have been brought on by an inherited genetic flaw, exposure to a toxin or virus, or both.

Exposure to specific viruses Certain childhood malignancies, such Hodgkin and non-Hodgkin lymphomas, have been associated to an increased chance of developing Epstein-Barr virus and HIV, the virus that causes AIDS. The virus may change a cell in some way. Following that, that cell divides to form an altered cell, which eventually develops into a cancer cell that divides to make even more cancer cells.

Environmental hazards. For a direct connection to childhood malignancies, research has been done on pesticides, fertilizers, and electrical lines. There is evidence that unrelated youngsters in particular neighborhoods and/or cities are developing cancer. It is unknown if exposure to these substances during pregnancy or as a newborn causes cancer or if it is just a coincidence.

Some kinds of radiation and high-dose chemotherapy. Children exposed to these agents may occasionally go on to acquire a second cancer later in life. These potent anticancer substances can change immune system components or cells. A second malignancy is a cancer that develops as a result of therapy for a primary malignancy.

Cancer Genes

How do genes impact cancer development?
An enormously significant advancement in the study of cancer has been the identification of certain gene types that contribute to the disease. It has been noted that over 90% of malignancies have some sort of genetic change. Some of these changes are

hereditary, while others are sporadic, which implies they happen by accident or result from exposure to the environment (usually over many years).

Cancer gene classifications

In certain types of cancer, three primary types of genes, including the following, are altered (mutated) and have the potential to effect cell growth:

- Oncogenes: These genes control a cell's proper growth. Oncogenes are usually described by scientists as being analogous to a cancer "switch" that most people have in their bodies. It is unknown what "flips the switch" that causes these oncogenes to suddenly lose their ability to regulate normal cell growth and start permitting aberrant cancer cells to thrive.
- Tumor suppressor genes: These genes can stop cancer cells' reproduction when they exhibit aberrant cell growth or division and can do so until the problem is fixed. However, tumor growth may happen if the tumor suppressor genes have been altered and are not functioning correctly.
- Mismatch-repair genes: These genes aid in spotting mistakes made during DNA cloning to create new cells. These genes fix the mismatch and correct the error if the DNA does not "match" precisely. However, if these genes are not functioning correctly, DNA mistakes may be passed on to future cells and harm them.

Normally, the number of cells in all of our bodily tissues is strictly regulated to ensure that both new cells and replacement cells are produced for healthy growth and development. Cancer is ultimately a loss of this equilibrium brought on by genetic changes that "tilt the scale" in favor of excessive cell development.

CHAPTER TWO
HEALTHY DIET

It's critical to comprehend some of the distinctive features of cancer metabolism in order to comprehend how diet can impact cancer treatment and prognosis. The Warburg effect, named after Otto Warburg, was his 1925 discovery that malignant tumors absorb more glucose than other tissues and utilize it without using oxidative phosphorylation. Although aerobic glycolysis produces less ATP than oxidative phosphorylation, it is thought to support cancer cell metabolism more effectively for a variety of reasons. First, a moderately hypoxic environment might result from tumors' potential for rapid growth, sometimes exceeding their blood supply. Second, because glycolysis does not require mitochondria and has a considerably smaller metabolic infrastructure than oxidative phosphorylation, it is more efficient. Third, the anapleurosis pathway can employ carbon atoms from glucose to create amino acids, nucleic acids, and other metabolic intermediates.

Over the past century, there has been a substantial advancement in our knowledge of the Warburg effect. It has been demonstrated that many cancer cells do have high respiratory rates, negating the need for aerobic metabolism in these cells. According to research by the Lisanti group, cancer cells cause stromal cells in their surroundings to switch to aerobic metabolism, releasing lactate and pyruvate that the cancer cells require for oxidative metabolism. The stromal cells are primarily responsible for this "Reverse Warburg Effect," which may lead to an overall increase in glucose absorption and aerobic metabolism in a tumor.

In addition to using more glucose, cancer cells frequently show a dependency on free fatty acids (FFA). FFA provide the acyl chains of phospholipids, which are the main building block of lipid bilayer membranes in cells and organelles. Every time a cell divides, its plasma membranes are duplicated, so for a cancer cell to multiply, a lot of FFA is needed. One molecule of palmitate requires 14 NADPH and 7 ATP, making FFA production an energy-intensive process. Both increased exogenous FFA absorption and increased de novo FFA synthesis have been linked to cancer aggressiveness and survival. FFA, on the other hand, can offer a significant amount of energy and are frequently present in tumor microenvironments, especially those close to adipocytes. Therefore, it has been demonstrated that cancer cells in adipocyte-rich settings rely substantially on FFA oxidation.

Amino acids can also be found in adipocytes. We have demonstrated that the L-asparaginase treatment of acute lymphoblastic leukemia can be significantly hampered by the release of glutamine and asparagine from adipocytes. Other cancer cells also depend heavily on glutamine because it helps them synthesize TCA cycle intermediates, nucleotides, and amino acids. The branched chain aminotransferase enzymes necessary for BCAA metabolism are frequently overexpressed by cancer cells, which require BCAAs for protein synthesis and energy metabolism. As a result, cancer cells have specific metabolic requirements that may be satisfied in situations where there is an abundance of adipose tissue.

Weight changes during cancer treatment

The body can experience significant changes in weight and composition both after the onset of cancer and during therapy. Cachexia, which involves weight loss that disproportionately affects lean body mass, is linked to a number of malignancies. Anorexia can be made worse by the pain, despair, and nausea connected to a cancer diagnosis and its therapies, whereas cachexia is typically related to inflammatory cytokines associated with cancer burden, such as TNF, IL-6, and IL-1α. Cachexia-related weight loss is typically regarded as a bad prognostic indicator. Cancer cachexia may indicate an aggressive or advanced form of the disease or a more severe reaction to therapy. Alternately (or furthermore), the unhealthily low weight associated with cachexia may potentially harm the effectiveness of cancer treatment.

On the other hand, some malignancies can cause significant weight gain over time. Due to the adipogenic properties of these drugs, tumors treated with high doses of glucocorticoids, especially hematologic cancers, are linked to a rise in adiposity. We demonstrated that, in adolescents receiving treatment for high-risk acute lymphoblastic leukemia (ALL), BMI was not a reliable indicator of obesity; over the course of the first month of the regimen, subjects gained 1.5 kg of body fat while losing 6 kg of lean mass, resulting in a significantly higher body fat percentage. Therefore, it was difficult to discern these changes in body fat using weight or BMI, and even people who lost weight frequently developed "sarcopenic obesity". Throughout ALL treatment, there is a risk for excess adiposity and obesity, and pediatric cancer survivors have a fourfold increased risk of developing metabolic syndrome, which includes obesity, hypertension, dyslipidemia, and insulin resistance.

During chemotherapy, the bone marrow environment also experiences significant alterations. The majority of chemotherapy drugs are toxic to hematopoietic cells, which causes a sharp decline in the amount of marrow space occupied by hematopoietic cells. Adipocytes fill a significant portion of this area through unknown ways. This is made worse by some cancer treatments that employ steroids, and the bone marrow in the long bones and iliac crest might change into tissue that is primarily made of fat. These fat cells might help hematologic and other malignancies that live in or spread to the marrow by encouraging their growth.

Dietary interventions

It is not surprising that dietary intervention has been a hot topic of discussion in the world of cancer treatment given the associations between obesity and poor cancer outcomes, the observation that cancer cells are excessive users of metabolic fuels like glucose, amino acids, and fats, and the strong desire of patients, families, and practitioners to offer further hope. Dietary therapies may improve results with little to no additional toxicity if they are shown to be favorable to therapy efficacy. In fact, some evidence suggest that dietary modifications may lessen the negative effects of chemotherapy. There aren't many food therapies that have been scientifically verified that can be offered to cancer patients, which is unfortunate because the great majority of the conversation has been based on opinion and anecdotal evidence. The preclinical and clinical research supporting the most popular dietary recommendations for cancer patients is summarized below.

Calorie limitation

Numerous preclinical research have examined the impact of caloric restriction on the development and progression of cancer, again with a wide range of cancer models, dietary interventions, and outcomes assessed. Most studies reduce calories by cutting back on carbohydrates, but some also limit protein or all nutrients proportionally. Animals are typically given between 60% and 85% of what an ad libitum (AL) control would eat when diet is imposed as a chronic condition. More severe calorie restriction, typically 50–67% of AL over 1-3 week intervals, is involved in intermittent methods. These restraint times are interspersed with intervals of either full AL consumption or AL group-matched consumption (to prevent compensatory overeating during nonfasting periods). As a result, comparing studies that employ various calorie restriction plans can be challenging.

Calorie restriction can delay cancer in spontaneous and carcinogenesis models as well as transplant in syngeneic and xenograft models, despite the variations in regimens. Studies that found caloric restriction to have no effect or a detrimental effect are few and few between. Several research have looked into whether caloric restriction can increase the effectiveness of treatment. Our research demonstrated that changing mice's diets from high-fat to low-fat boosted vincristine's effectiveness in treating syngeneic B-cell ALL; however, we found no synergy with dexamethasone or L-asparaginase.

Ketogenic diet/carbohydrate restriction

The use of a ketogenic diet as an alternative to fasting and calorie restriction has garnered a lot of attention. Some people may handle a ketogenic diet better than others, and it has a long history of safety as an epilepsy treatment. A recent meta-analysis of 12 research that compared an unrestricted ketogenic diet to a regular diet in murine cancer models found that the ketogenic diet generally caused development to be delayed. A few studies have examined the effectiveness of a ketogenic diet during anti-cancer therapy, finding that chemotherapy, metformin, and radiation therapy frequently work in synergy.

Six studies describing clinical ketogenic diet intervention in pediatric or adult glioma patients, collectively encompassing 39 people, were found in a recent systematic review, along with 12 ongoing trials. The results indicated that a ketogenic diet could be well-tolerated with few side effects and may confer some benefit to overall and progression free survival, despite the fact that none of the published studies were randomized control trials. However, the case-series study designs without comparisons to control groups preclude more conclusive conclusions.

Additional dietary strategies

Numerous diets that don't fall into the aforementioned categories have been found to have positive effects on cancer risk and prognosis. Strict adherence to a Mediterranean diet has been linked to decreased mortality from all causes of cancer, as well as breast, colorectal, head and neck, gastric, prostate, liver, pulmonary, and pancreatic cancer mortality. The Mediterranean diet includes a lot of olive oil, which has high levels of MUFA, antioxidants, and other nutrients that may be helpful. The likelihood of developing breast, gastrointestinal, and general cancer was lower in those who consumed the most olive oil. Although reduced animal protein intake was not linked to a higher risk of dying from cancer in prospective cohorts, protein restriction can slow the growth of human xenograft breast and prostate tumors. According to a meta-analysis of 96 cohort and cross-sectional studies, eating a vegetarian or vegan diet decreased the risk of developing cancer by 8% and 15%, respectively. Following a prostate cancer diagnosis, a higher diet of vegetable rather than animal fats was linked to a better survival rate. Increased soy consumption was linked in a meta-analysis to a lower risk of breast death and recurrence. Numerous studies have examined individual dietary elements for their potential to fight cancer in both in vitro and preclinical settings (for example,). To our knowledge, no studies have been done to determine whether any of these diets or dietary components can enhance the effectiveness of chemotherapy treatment.

Which diet is best for cancer therapy?

Preclinical research can teach us a lot about obesity, food, and cancer prognosis, but it's crucial to remember that mice are not humans. The food-induced obese C57BL/6 mice, the most widely used rodent model of obesity, develops obesity on a diet that contains 45% to 60% of calories from fat. In contrast, obesity is regarded to be more closely associated with excess carbs in humans. Few studies have compared different diets head-to-head, and even when they do, the "winning" diet may be superior merely because of the particulars of the models used. For instance, caloric restriction at 60% of ad libitum improved survival in p53 heterozygous mice more than weekly fasting. But what if they had experimented with fasting every other day or twice a week? In order to protect mice against doxorubicin toxicity, a 60-hour fast was more successful than a 50% caloric restriction (22), but what if it wasn't as effective at enhancing its anti-cancer activity? Or with the function of an alternative chemotherapy? In these kinds of studies, it is challenging, if not impossible, to compare "fair" diets because matching calorie intake does not always equate to tolerance. Additionally, diets may behave differently in various cancer models depending on the kind, stage, mutations, species, treatment plan, etc. of the cancer. In a recent meta-analysis, the effectiveness of intermittent calorie restriction was found to be superior than chronic calorie restriction for carcinogen models and more successful in reducing the incidence of cancer in genetically modified models (30). It is challenging to convert these findings into clinical advice.

The effectiveness of caloric restriction, the ketogenic diet, and intermittent fasting on cancer initiation, progression, and metastasis were compared in a systematic review and meta-analysis that included many of the studies mentioned above; the authors came to the conclusion that caloric restriction and the ketogenic diet were highly effective, while the data on intermittent fasting were not yet conclusive. More research will be required to determine which nutritional treatments are most effective in treating various diseases because there is a dearth of information about how they affect cancer patients.

Our diet clearly has a significant impact on our risk of developing cancer. The potential of nutrition management to enhance cancer treatment results is well supported by the preclinical literature. The ideal dietary approach is not yet known, and it is anticipated that the effectiveness of a diet will vary depending on the patient, the kind of cancer, and the course of treatment. When implementing these tactics in the clinic, some personalization may be required because doctors who treat overweight and obese patients are aware that sometimes the best diet is the one the patient is willing and able to follow. Unfortunately, this calls for adaptability, auxiliary support personnel, and awareness that a lifestyle intervention may be as effective as cytotoxic drugs.

Although it is difficult to apply these findings from mice to people, we must keep looking into this possibility. Dietary changes could lead to a better prognosis for cancer patients without adding any new toxins or long-term consequences. In fact, the majority of the research suggests that changing one's diet can lower toxicity and make chemotherapy more effective. The integration of this paradigm shift into oncology will take additional time and clinical studies.

CHAPTER THREE

FASTING

Fasting is the practice of going without food for an extended period of time or taking extremely few calories. The duration of a fasting cycle might range from 12 hours to 3 weeks.

According to numerous studies, both short and long fasting periods have positive effects on the treatment and prevention of cancer. However, it is yet unknown which fasting schedule yields the greatest outcomes.

Fasting may be beneficial in cancer therapy. A growing number of research is showing the benefits of fasting for both treating and preventing cancer.

According to several studies, fasting reduces insulin resistance and levels of inflammation, which may help the body fight cancer. Chronic diseases like obesity and type 2 diabetes, which are both risk factors for cancer, may be reversed by fasting as well.

Additionally, according to studies, fasting may protect healthy cells while increasing the chemotherapeutic response of cancer cells. Fasting may also strengthen the immune system and aid in the battle against already-existing cancer.

The effects of fasting on the treatment and prevention of cancer are discussed in this chapter.

Increasing Sensitivity to Insulin

A hormone called insulin enables cells to take up glucose from the blood and use it as fuel.

The body's cells become less responsive to insulin when there is a greater supply of food available. Because of this insulin resistance, cells no longer react to insulin signals, which raises blood glucose levels and increases fat accumulation.

The human body makes an effort to conserve as much energy as it can when food is in short supply.

It does this through increasing the sensitivity of cell membranes to insulin, among other things. Insulin can remove glucose from the blood more effectively in cells than in tissues.

Better insulin sensitivity inhibits the growth and development of cancer cells.

Reversing the effects of chronic diseases

According to some studies, cancer risk factors include diseases like type 2 diabetes and obesity. Both have been connected to reduced survival rates and a higher chance of developing various cancers.

In a case study published in 2017, the impact of brief fasting on type 2 diabetes was examined. Two to three times a week, the study subject fasted for 24 hours.

The participant's weight was down 17.8% and their waist size was down 11% after 4 months of fasting.

Additionally, after two months of this fasting pattern, they were no longer in need of insulin therapy.

Enhancing Autophagy

Cellular processes called autophagy allow for the breakdown of cell components for eventual re-use. Autophagy is essential for preserving healthy cell function and aids in the defense of bodily cells. Cancer prevention and treatment benefit greatly from the activity of autophagy.

Several mouse studies indicate that autophagy may guard against cancer. These investigations demonstrate that tumor-suppressing genes are expressed at lower levels when autophagy is absent.

Lower autophagy may facilitate the initial development of tumors, but it is not the only factor in the growth or spread of malignant tumors.

Improving Living Conditions While Receiving Chemotherapy

According to some researchers, fasting enhances a person's reaction to chemotherapy because it:

- stimulates cellular renewal

- lowers the impact of side effects such fatigue, nausea, headaches, and cramping
- protects blood against the damaging effects of chemotherapy

According to a 2018 study, fasting can enhance quality of life in patients receiving chemotherapy for ovarian or breast cancer. A 60-hour fasting period beginning 36 hours before the start of chemotherapy treatment was used in the study.

The findings demonstrate that participants who fasted during chemotherapy experienced improved chemotolerance, less side effects associated with chemo, and higher energy levels in comparison to those who did not fast.

Increasing Immunity to Fight Cancer

In a 2014 study, researchers looked at whether mouse stem cells could be used to fight cancer. Because of their capacity for regeneration, stem cells are significant.

According to the study, fasting for two to four days may shield stem cells from the damaging effects of chemotherapy on the immune system.

Additionally, fasting stimulates immune system stem cells to regenerate and repair themselves.

This study demonstrates that fasting not only lessens cell damage but also refills and replaces damaged white blood cells.

White blood cells eliminate potentially harmful cells and combat infection. Chemotherapy lowers white blood cell counts, which has a deleterious impact on the immune system. As a result, the body struggles more to combat infections.

Fasting causes the body's white blood cell count to drop. White blood cell levels rise when the fasting period is over and the body starts taking in food.

CHAPTER FOUR
EXERCISE

Exercise is an essential part of cancer treatment. Numerous studies indicate that regular exercise can significantly enhance both physical and mental health during all stages of treatment. Even if you weren't active before your cancer diagnosis, you may get moving safely and effectively with the aid of a fitness program that is tailored to your specific needs.

What advantages does exercise provide for cancer patients?

Exercise with cancer treatment has various advantages. A few of these are:

Enhance the efficacy of treatment and lessen adverse effects. In general, regardless of the stage or kind of cancer, exercise can enhance the body's reaction to treatment. Exercise regularly has been demonstrated to:

- lessen weariness brought on by treatment
- Maintain physical capability, strength, and heart and lung health.
- may improve quality of life and lessen symptoms of anxiety and despair.

- Reduce the amount of hospital recuperation time required following lung cancer surgery.

Exercise has also been linked in certain studies to higher survival rates for specific cancers, such as colorectal and breast cancer.

Enhance general state of health. Exercise can generally benefit a patient's overall health. Exercise has a variety of health advantages, including:

- Boost your balance to lower your risk of falling.
- remaining as independent and mobile as possible
- halt muscle deterioration and increase strength
- Help with weight loss or maintenance
- enhance sleep
- Osteoporosis risk should be reduced

lower the risk of other malignancies and co-existing diseases. In addition to cancer, you may also experience co-existing diseases. Consistent exercise may:

- decrease the likelihood of co-occurring diseases like diabetes and heart disease developing
- assist you in managing any existing coexisting conditions.
- decrease the likelihood of getting more malignancies

Enhance mental health. It has been demonstrated that exercise lowers the chances of anxiety and depression.

Things you need to know before you exercise during cancer therapy

Before beginning an exercise regimen during or after cancer treatment, always consult your doctor. If you exercised regularly before therapy, you might or might not be able to continue doing so while you are getting treatment.

It will take some time to get back to your pre-cancer fitness level after treatment. Your healthcare staff can advise you on the best workout regimen for you. They may give you the go-ahead to begin working out independently, or they may recommend a cancer rehabilitation program or a certified cancer exercise specialist who can create the ideal exercise plan for your particular circumstances. You might be able to stick to the plan on your own, or you might need to spend some time working with the cancer rehabilitation clinician or exercise specialist. Your specific fitness program will be based on:

- the kind of your cancer
- The procedures being utilized
- The negative consequences you're going through
- Your degree of exercise
- Any further medical conditions you may have

Developing your exercise regimen

The American Society of Clinical Oncology (ASCO) advises cancer patients to engage in aerobic and strength-training exercise while undergoing cancer therapy based on the body of knowledge. ASCO does not currently advocate a specific type or amount of exercise to lessen the side effects of cancer treatment due to a lack of adequate research on exercise during cancer treatment.

The following material gives a summary of exercise suggestions that have been demonstrated to enhance overall health and may be taken into account before and after cancer treatment.

Stretching. Regular stretching helps enhance posture and flexibility. Your body can heal itself thanks to the increased blood and oxygen supply to the muscles. If you haven't been active while recovering from cancer treatments, stretching can be quite beneficial. For instance, radiation therapy can reduce your range of motion and make your muscles stiff, but regular stretching both before and after can help you move more freely and remain flexible. Stretching after surgery can aid in reducing tight scar tissue and regaining range of motion, allowing you to resume your normal daily activities.

Balance training. A side effect of cancer and its treatment is balance loss. Exercises that improve your balance will help you restore the mobility and function you need to resume your regular activities in a safe manner. Keeping your equilibrium also helps you avoid accidents like falls.

Aerobic Exercise. Cardio is another name for this sort of exercise, which increases heart rate. It can make you feel less exhausted both during and after treatment because it strengthens the heart and lungs of the body. It's simple to gain cardio exercise by walking. For instance, your medical staff might advise doing moderately paced walks for 40 to 50 minutes, three to four times each week.

Exercising your muscles. When a person is less active throughout cancer treatment and recuperation, muscle loss frequently occurs. Muscle weakness might also result from some treatments. You may keep and develop strong muscles by engaging in resistance exercise, often known as strength training. Gaining muscle mass might help you balance better, feel less worn out, and find it simpler to perform regular tasks. Additionally, it can aid in the fight against osteoporosis, a bone thinning condition brought on by several cancer treatments.

Two days per week of full-body strength exercise are advised by the Centers for Disease Control and Prevention (CDC) in the United States. Exercise equipment, resistance bands, hand weights, and your own body weight can all be used in a strength training regimen.

How to work out while receiving cancer therapy safely

Exercise safety measures are crucial if you are experiencing side effects from cancer or its treatment. Depending on the precise side effects you experience, you might need to modify your workout regimen. For instance, using weight machines rather than hand weights may be safer if your treatment is damaging the nerves in your hands. Ask about avoiding neck-straining workouts that increase the risk of falling if your treatment has caused bone loss.

Here are some additional tips to help you maximize your exercise program safely:

- Begin gradually. Even if you were physically active prior to receiving cancer treatment, gradually increase your exercise level. This can help you avoid harm and prevent discouragement.
- Exercise in a secure setting. Avoid huge gyms where germs can readily spread if your immune system has been compromised by therapy. If it's nice outside, exercise outside or at home.
- Be aware of your body. If you don't feel like exercising because you lack energy, reduce the time or intensity until you do.
- Keep hydrated and consume a balanced diet. To prevent dehydration, consume enough of water throughout the day and during your workouts. Consuming wholesome foods, particularly those strong in protein, aids in your body's

post-workout recovery. You can create a nutrition plan with the aid of an oncology nutritionist.
- Visit your physician frequently. Your health may deteriorate during and following therapy. During your routine checkups, discuss your vital health metrics with your doctor to determine whether it is safe for you to exercise. These metrics may include your blood count.

How does exercise fit into a regimen for cancer rehabilitation?

Exercise is occasionally used in cancer recovery programs. It's critical to comprehend the distinction between physical activity and cancer rehabilitation. A person can restore or retain their capacity to perform while receiving cancer therapy by participating in a thorough treatment program known as cancer rehabilitation. Before being able to safely exercise alone, a person with cancer may occasionally need cancer rehabilitation to regain their strength and balance. The therapies utilized to address particular health and mobility difficulties are the exercises that are a part of a comprehensive cancer rehabilitation plan.

Ask your medical staff if speaking with a cancer rehabilitation specialist will be beneficial for you.

Ask the medical staff these questions

Consider posing the following inquiries to your medical staff:

- What sort of fitness regimen would you suggest for me?
- Could this workout routine evolve over time?
- Do I need to refrain from doing any particular exercises while receiving cancer treatment? What happens when my medical therapy is over?
- Do you advise me to seek cancer rehabilitation?
- Does my cancer treatment require me to forgo going to the gym? What kinds of exercises can I do at home, if so?

CHAPTER FIVE
REGULAR CHECK-UPS

We cannot ease the focus on prevention, treatment, and care for communicable diseases because they continue to be the leading causes of death in the world today, including HIV/AIDS, tuberculosis, and diarrheal illnesses. Non-communicable diseases (NCDs), which are illnesses or ailments that are not contagious but are the cause of early death and poor health, have increased significantly in the meantime. Heart conditions, diabetes, and cancer are a few of the chronic NCDs. Interactions between communicable and non-communicable diseases can potentially be fatal. HPV and hepatitis B and C infections "substantially contribute to the burden of [the WHO Africa region's] top two cancers," which are liver and cervical cancer, according to the World Health Organization. Additionally, having HIV raises a person's chance of cervical cancer. Therefore, we cannot prioritize one category of disorders over another. The diets of people are changing, and not for the better, as the world urbanizes. People who relocate to cities run the risk of being exposed to carcinogens in the environment, unhealthy and unregulated meals, and dangerous substances like alcohol and smoke.

Cancer is one of the most prevalent NCDs. It is now uncommon to meet someone whose life has not been affected by it. Two-thirds of cancer fatalities, according to the WHO, take place in low- and middle-income nations.

Unfortunately, if treatment is to be effective, diagnosis is sometimes made too late. Knowing your position is essential for this reason. Fortunately, effective public health initiatives have raised awareness of HIV status to the point where it is now expected. The duty to safeguard our own and our loved ones' health does not, however, end there.

Life expectancy has grown as a result of recent considerable improvements in the public health environment on the globe. Since then, there have been fewer cases of infectious diseases and longer lifespans. The likelihood of having non-communicable diseases rises as people live longer.

Why should you be aware of your cancer status?

With 8.2 million mortalities attributed to it in 2012, cancer ranked among the top causes of morbidity and mortality worldwide. In the following two decades, this number is predicted to nearly double. One of the top four NCDs today is cancer.

Early cancer detection often leads to successful treatment. Early detection and appropriate care are crucial and required. The majority of cancer-related deaths can be avoided, particularly if the early warning signals are recognized and promptly managed. The suggested age for screening for those at typical risk must be performed earlier for those with a family history of cancer.

Various cancer screening procedures are advised depending on the patient's age, gender, and family history.

Cancer is the third most common cause of death in Kenya, after cardiovascular and infectious disorders. A significant share of cancer victims are under the age of 70, according to the Kenya National Cancer Control Strategy (2017-2022). Cervical, breast, and esophageal cancer in women are the most prevalent kinds of the disease. The most common cancers in men are Kaposi sarcoma, esophageal, and prostate. Women should begin breast cancer screening at the age of 40, and males should begin prostate cancer screening at the age of 50. Testing is advised early if there is a family history of cancer. As early as age 21, testing for cervical cancer is advised.

You cannot afford to avoid cancer screening.

The simplest approaches to guarantee prompt treatment beginning are screening and early detection. For those who are a specific age or have a family history of cancer, these screens might be incorporated into routine examinations. Due to the National Health Insurance Fund's expansion of medical coverage to cancer patients, all Kenyans now have access to cancer care and treatment.

Regular cancer screenings and prompt treatment initiation are crucial. Governments at the county and federal levels ought to think about organizing public screenings in underserved areas. Additionally, they should pledge to intensify and broaden public education about NCDs, including cancer, in lower-level medical facilities.

Finally, being aware of your cancer status is similar to being aware of the state of any other illness. A cancer diagnosis does not automatically mean death. Cancer patients can be cured, continue working, and live long lives.

CONCLUSION

Over the past ten years, early identification and curative treatments have greatly increased the number of cancer survivors and improved management and lifestyle choices. Despite the rise in survival rates, many survivors continue to live in constant anxiety of a recurrence or the appearance of a new comorbidity.

Survivors are more likely to die from non-cancer related reasons, particularly cardio-respiratory illnesses, than from second primary malignancies or cancer recurrence.

Survivorship treatment includes both medical and mental concerns. In order to guarantee that cancer survivors receive thorough survivorship care, it is imperative that all aspects of care are given careful consideration. Healthy lifestyle choices like a balanced diet, frequent exercise, and fasting have the power to significantly lower morbidity and mortality rates in cancer survivors. Successful weight control has also been linked to a reduction in chronic or recurrent disorders, according to research.

After treatment, survivors can regain strength by consuming a diet rich in fruits, vegetables, and unprocessed low-fat meals. Experts advise eating lean proteins and plant-based diets. Their odds of developing diabetes, obesity, high blood pressure, and heart problems can be decreased by eating healthfully.

By adopting current health recommendations and encouraging patients to actively participate in pursuing general preventive health initiatives, care providers can help their patients.

www.ingramcontent.com/pod-product-compliance
Lightning Source LLC
Chambersburg PA
CBHW050320220526
45465CB00005B/2058